RENAL DIET

Kidney Diet Cookbook for Beginners Low Sodium - Potassium and Phosphorus Recipes for Healthy Cook's Kitchen with Diet Food Plan

TABLE OF CONTENTS

BREAKFAST

Egg and Veggie Muffins

Preparation Time: 15 minutes

Cooking Time: 20 minutes

Servings: 4

Ingredients:

- 4 Eggs

- 2 Tbsp. Unsweetened rice milk

- ½ chopped Sweet onion

- ½ chopped Red bell pepper

- Pinch red pepper flakes

- Pinch ground black pepper

Directions:

1. Preheat the oven to 350F.

2. Spray 4 muffin pans with cooking spray. Set aside.

3. Whisk the milk, eggs, onion, red pepper, parsley, red pepper flakes, and black pepper until mixed.

4. Pour the egg mixture into prepared muffin pans.

5. Bake until the muffins are puffed and golden, about 18 to 20 minutes. Serve.

Nutrition: Calories: 84 Fat: 5g Carb: 3g Protein: 7g Sodium: 75mg Potassium: 117mg Phosphorus: 110mg

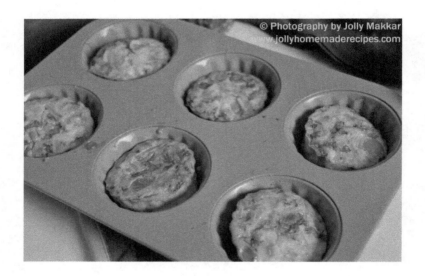

Berry Chia with Yogurt

Preparation Time: 35 minutes

Cooking Time: 5 minutes

Servings:4

Ingredients:

- ½ cup chia seeds, dried
- 2 cup Plain yogurt
- 1/3 cup strawberries, chopped
- ¼ cup blackberries
- ¼ cup raspberries
- 4 teaspoons Splenda

Directions:

1. Mix up together Plain yogurt with Splenda, and chia seeds.
2. Transfer the mixture into the serving ramekins (jars) and leave for 35 minutes.
3. After this, add blackberries, raspberries, and strawberries. Mix up the meal well.
4. Serve it immediately or store it in the fridge for up to 2 days.

Nutrition: Calories: 150 Fat: 5g Carbs: 19g Protein: 6.8g Sodium: 65mg Potassium: 226mg Phosphorus: 75mg

Arugula Eggs with Chili Peppers

Preparation Time: 7 minutes

Cooking Time: 10 minutes

Servings: 4

Ingredients:

- 2 cups arugula, chopped
- 3 eggs, beaten
- ½ chili pepper, chopped
- 1 tablespoon butter
- 1 oz Parmesan, grated

Directions:

1. Toss butter in the skillet and melt it.
2. Add arugula and sauté it over medium heat for 5 minutes. Stir it from time to time.
3. Meanwhile, mix up together Parmesan, chili pepper, and eggs.
4. Pour the egg mixture over the arugula and scramble well.
5. Cook for 5 minutes more over medium heat.

Nutrition: Calories: 218 Fat: 15g Carbs: 2.8g Protein: 17g Sodium: 656mg Potassium: 243mg Phosphorus: 310mg

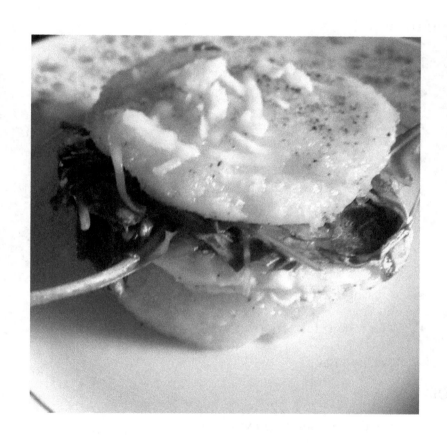

Eggplant Chicken Sandwich

Preparation Time: 10 minutes

Cooking Time: 15 minutes

Servings: 2

Ingredients:

- 1 eggplant, trimmed

- 10 oz chicken fillet

- 1 teaspoon Plain yogurt

- ½ teaspoon minced garlic

- 1 tablespoon fresh cilantro, chopped

- 2 lettuce leaves

- 1 teaspoon olive oil

- ½ teaspoon salt

- ½ teaspoon chili pepper

- 1 teaspoon butter

Directions:

1. Slice the eggplant lengthwise into 4 slices.

2. Rub the eggplant slices with minced garlic and brush with olive oil.

3. Grill the eggplant slices on the preheated to 375F grill for 3 minutes from each side.

4. Meanwhile, rub the chicken fillet with salt and chili pepper.

5. Place it in the skillet and add butter.

6. Roast the chicken for 6 minutes from each side over medium-high heat.

7. Cool the cooked eggplants gently and spread one side of them with Plain yogurt.

8. Add lettuce leaves and chopped fresh cilantro.

9. After this, slice the cooked chicken fillet and add over the lettuce.

10. Cover it with the remaining sliced eggplant to get the sandwich shape. Pin the sandwich with the toothpick if needed.

Nutrition: Calories: 276 Fat: 11g Carbs: 41g Protein: 13.8g Sodium: 775mg Potassium: 532mg Phosphorus: 187mg

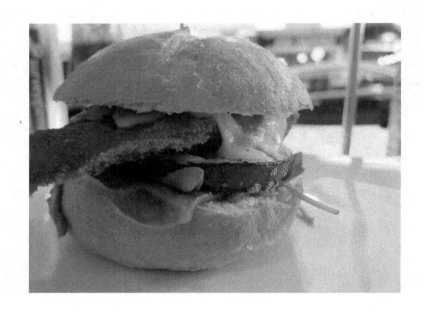

Apple Pumpkin Muffins

Preparation time: 15 minutes

Cooking time: 20 minutes

Servings: 12

Ingredients

- 1 cup all-purpose flour
- 1 cup wheat bran
- 2 teaspoons phosphorus powder
- 1 cup pumpkin purée
- ¼ cup honey
- ¼ cup olive oil
- 1 egg
- 1 teaspoon vanilla extract
- ½ cup cored diced apple

Directions

1. Preheat the oven to 400°f.

2. Line 12 muffin cups with paper liners.

3. Stir together the flour, wheat bran, and baking powder, mix this in a medium bowl.

4. In a small bowl, whisk together the pumpkin, honey, olive oil, egg, and vanilla.

5. Stir the pumpkin mixture into the flour mixture until just combined.

6. Stir in the diced apple.

7. Spoon the batter in the muffin cups.

8. Bake for about 20 minutes, or until a toothpick inserted in the center of a muffin comes out clean.

Nutrition per serving: (1 muffin): calories: 125; total fat: 5g; saturated fat: 1g; cholesterol: 18mg; sodium: 8mg; carbohydrates: 20g; fiber: 3g; phosphorus: 120mg; potassium: 177mg; protein: 2g

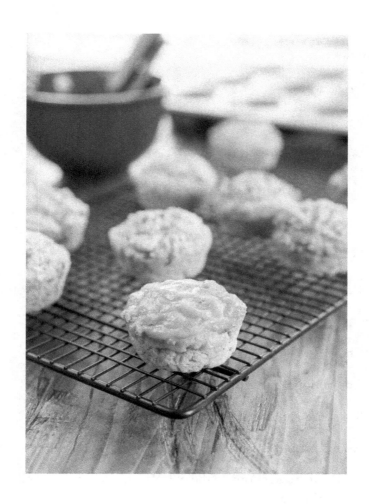

Chorizo Bowl with Corn

Preparation Time: 10 minutes

Cooking Time: 15 minutes

Servings: 4

Ingredients:

- 9 oz chorizo
- 1 tablespoon almond butter
- ½ cup corn kernels
- ¾ cup heavy cream
- 1 teaspoon butter
- ¼ teaspoon chili pepper
- 1 tablespoon dill, chopped

Directions:

1. Chop the chorizo and place it in the skillet.
2. Add almond butter and chili pepper.
3. Roast the chorizo for 3 minutes.
4. After this, add corn kernels.
5. Add butter and chopped the dill. Mix up the mixture well—Cook for 2 minutes.
6. Close the lid and simmer for 10 minutes over low heat.
7. Transfer the cooked meal into the serving bowls.

Nutrition: Calories: 286 Fat: 15g Carbs: 26g Protein: 13g Sodium: 228mg Potassium: 255mg Phosphorus: 293mg

Panzanella Salad

Preparation Time: 10 minutes

Cooking Time: 5 minutes

Servings: 4

Ingredients:

- 2 cucumbers, chopped

- 1 red onion, sliced

- 2 red bell peppers, chopped

- ¼ cup fresh cilantro, chopped

- 1 tablespoon capers

- 1 oz whole-grain bread, chopped

- 1 tablespoon canola oil

- ½ teaspoon minced garlic

- 1 tablespoon Dijon mustard

- 1 teaspoon olive oil

- 1 teaspoon lime juice

Directions:

1. Pour canola oil into the skillet and bring it to boil.

2. Add chopped bread and roast it until crunchy (3-5 minutes).

3. Meanwhile, in the salad bowl, combine sliced red onion, cucumbers, bell peppers, cilantro, capers, and mix up gently.

4. Make the dressing: mix up together lime juice, olive oil, Dijon mustard, and minced garlic.

5. Put the dressing over the salad and stir it directly before serving.

Nutrition: Calories: 224.3 Fat: 10g Carbs: 26g Protein: 6.6g Sodium: 401mg Potassium: 324.9mg Phosphorus: 84mg

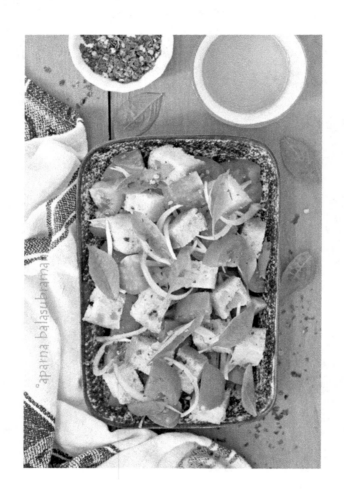

LUNCH

Green Palak Paneer

Preparation Time: 5 minutes

Cooking Time: 10 minutes

Servings: 4

Ingredients:

- 1-pound green lettuce
- 2 cups cubed paneer (vegan)
- 2 tablespoons coconut oil
- 1 teaspoon cumin
- 1 chopped up onion
- 1-2 teaspoons hot green chili minced up
- 1 teaspoon minced garlic
- 15 cashews
- 4 tablespoons almond milk
- 1 teaspoon Garam masala
- Flavored vinegar as needed

Directions:

1. Add cashews and almond milk to a blender and blend well.
2. Set your pot to Sauté mode and add coconut oil; allow the oil to heat up.
3. Add cumin seeds, garlic, green chilies, ginger and sauté for 1 minute.
4. Add onion and sauté for 2 minutes.
5. Add chopped green lettuce, flavored vinegar and a cup of water.

6. Lock up the lid and cook on HIGH pressure for 10 minutes.
7. Quick-release the pressure.
8. Add ½ cup of water and blend to a paste.
9. Add cashew paste, paneer and Garam Masala and stir thoroughly.
10. Serve over hot rice!

Nutrition: Calories: 367 Fat: 26g Carbohydrates: 21g Protein: 16g Phosphorus: 110mg Potassium: 117mg Sodium: 75mg

Cucumber Sandwich

Preparation Time: 1 hour

Cooking Time: 5 minutes

Servings: 2

Ingredients:

- 6 tsp. of cream cheese

- 1 pinch of dried dill weed

- 3 tsp. of mayonnaise

- .25 tsp. dry Italian dressing mix

- 4 slices of white bread

- .5 of a cucumber

Directions:

1. Prepare the cucumber and cut it into slices.

2. Mix cream cheese, mayonnaise, and Italian dressing. Chill for one hour.

3. Distribute the mixture onto the white bread slices.

4. Place cucumber slices on top and sprinkle with the dill weed.

5. Cut in halves and serve.

Nutrition: Calories: 143 Fat: 6g Carbs: 16.7g Protein: 4g Sodium: 255mg Potassium: 127mg Phosphorus: 64mg

Pizza Pitas

Preparation Time: 10 minutes

Cooking Time: 10 minutes

Servings: 1

Ingredients:

- .33 cup of mozzarella cheese

- 2 pieces of pita bread, 6 inches in size

- 6 tsp. of chunky tomato sauce

- 2 cloves of garlic (minced)

- .25 cups of onion, chopped small

- .25 tsp. of red pepper flakes

- .25 cup of bell pepper, chopped small

- 2 ounces of ground pork, lean

- No-stick oil spray

- .5 tsp. of fennel seeds

Directions:

1. Preheat oven to 400.

2. Put the garlic, ground meat, pepper flakes, onion, and bell pepper in a pan. Sauté until cooked.

3. Grease a flat baking pan and put pitas on it. Use the mixture to spread on the pita bread.

4. Spread one tablespoon of the tomato sauce and top with cheese.

5. Bake for five to eight minutes, until the cheese is bubbling.

Nutrition: Calories: 284 Fat: 10g Carbs: 34g Protein: 16g Sodium: 795mg Potassium: 706mg Phosphorus: 416mg

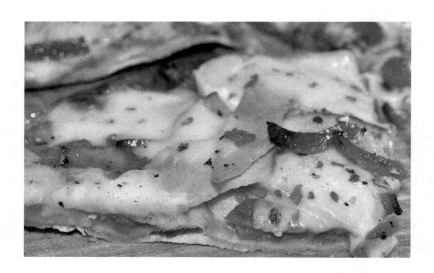

Lettuce Wraps with Chicken

Preparation Time: 10 minutes

Cooking Time: 15 minutes

Servings: 4

Ingredients:

- 8 lettuce leaves

- .25 cups of fresh cilantro

- .25 cups of mushroom

- 1 tsp. of five spices seasoning

- .25 cups of onion

- 6 tsp. of rice vinegar

- 2 tsp. of hoisin

- 6 tsp. of oil (canola)

- 3 tsp. of oil (sesame)

- 2 tsp. of garlic

- 2 scallions

- 8 ounces of cooked chicken breast

Directions:

1. Mince together the cooked chicken and the garlic. Chop up the onions, cilantro, mushrooms, and scallions.

2. Use a skillet overheat, combine chicken to all remaining ingredients, minus the lettuce leaves. Cook for fifteen minutes, stirring occasionally.

3. Place .25 cups of the mixture into each leaf of lettuce.

4. Wrap the lettuce around like a burrito and eat.

Nutrition: Calories: 84 Fat: 4g Carbs: 9g Protein: 5.9g Sodium: 618mg Potassium: 258mg Phosphorus: 64mg

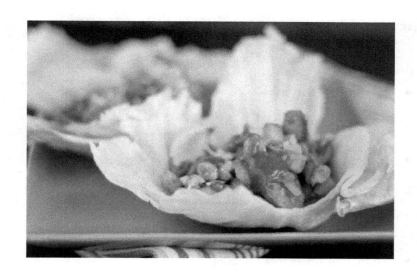

DINNER

Pork Meatloaf

Preparation Time: 10 minutes

Cooking Time: 50 minutes

Servings: 1

Ingredients:

- 1-pound lean ground beef
- ½ cup Breadcrumbs
- ½ cup Chopped sweet onion
- 1 Egg
- 2 tbsps. Chopped fresh basil
- 1 tsp. Chopped fresh thyme
- 1 tsp. Chopped fresh parsley
- ¼ tsp. Ground black pepper
- 1 tbsp. Brown sugar
- 1 tsp. White vinegar
- ¼ tsp. Garlic powder

Directions:

1. Preheat the oven to 350f.

2. Mix well the breadcrumbs, beef, onion, basil, egg, thyme, parsley, and pepper.

3. Stir the brown sugar, vinegar, and garlic powder in a small bowl.

4. Put the brown sugar mixture evenly over the meat.

5. Bake the meatloaf for about 50 minutes or until it is cooked through.

6. Let the meatloaf stand for 10 minutes and then pour out any accumulated grease.

Nutrition: Calories: 103 Fat: 3g Carb: 7g Protein: 11g Sodium: 87mg Potassium: 190mg Phosphorus: 112mg

Chicken Stew

Preparation Time: 20 minutes

Cooking Time: 50 minutes

Servings: 1

Ingredients:

- 1 tbsp. Olive oil
- 1 pound, cut into 1-inch cubes Boneless, skinless chicken thighs
- ½, chopped Sweet onion
- 1 tbsp. Minced garlic
- 2 cups Chicken stock
- 1 cup, plus 2 tbsps. Water
- 1 sliced Carrot
- 2 stalks, sliced Celery
- 1, sliced thin Turnip
- 1 tbsp. Chopped fresh thyme
- 1 tsp. Chopped fresh rosemary
- 2 tsp. Cornstarch
- Ground black pepper to taste

Directions:

1. Prepare a large saucepan on medium heat and add the olive oil.

2. Sauté the chicken for 6 minutes or until it is lightly browned, stirring often.

3. Add the onion and garlic, and sauté for 3 minutes.

4. Add 1-cup water, chicken stock, carrot, celery, and turnip and bring the stew to a boil.

5. Simmer for 30 minutes or until cooked and tender.

6. Add the thyme and rosemary and simmer for 3 minutes more.

7. In a small bowl, stir together the 2 tbsps. Of water and the cornstarch

8. add the mixture to the stew.

9. Stir to incorporate the cornstarch mixture and cook for 3 to 4 minutes or until the stew thickens.

10. Remove from the heat once done and season with pepper.

Nutrition: Calories: 141 Fat: 8g Carb: 5g Protein: 9g Sodium: 214mg Potassium: 192mg Phosphorus: 53mg

Apple & Cinnamon Spiced Honey Pork Loin

Preparation time: 20 minutes

Cooking time: 6 hours

Servings: 6

Ingredients

- 1 2-3lb boneless pork loin roast
- ½ teaspoon low-sodium salt
- ¼ teaspoon pepper
- 1 tablespoon canola oil
- 3 medium apples, peeled and sliced
- ¼ cup honey
- 1 small red onion, halved and sliced
- 1 tablespoon ground cinnamon

Directions

1. Season the pork with salt and pepper.
2. Heat the oil in a skillet and brown the pork on all sides.
3. Arrange half the apples in the base of a 4 to 6-quart slow cooker.
4. Top with the honey and remaining apples.
5. Sprinkle with cinnamon and cover.
6. Cover and cook on low for 6-8 hours until the meat is tender.

Nutrition: Calories 290, Fat 10g, Carbs 19g, Protein 29g, Fiber 2g, Potassium 789mg, Sodium 22mg

MAIN DISHES

Mushroom Crêpes

Preparation Time: 1 hour 30 minutes

Cooking Time: 30 minutes

Servings: 6

Ingredients:

- 2 eggs
- 3/4 cup almond milk
- 1/2 cup all-purpose flour
- 1/4 teaspoon salt
- For the filling
- 3 tablespoons all-purpose flour
- 2 cups of cremini mushrooms, sliced
- 3/4 cup chicken broth
- 1/2 cup Parmesan cheese, grated
- 1/8 teaspoon cayenne
- 1/8 teaspoon nutmeg
- ¾ cup almond milk
- 3 garlic cloves, minced
- 2 tablespoons of parsley (chopped)
- 6 slices of deli-sliced cooked lean ham
- 1/4 teaspoon of salt
- Freshly ground pepper

Directions:

1. Put and combine the salt and flour in a bowl. In another bowl, whisk the eggs and almond milk. Gradually combine the two mixtures until smooth. Leave for 15 minutes.
2. Spray a skillet using non-stick cooking spray and put over medium heat. Stir the batter a little. Add 1/4 of the batter into the skillet. Tilt the skillet to form a thin and even crêpe. Cook for 1-2 minutes or until the bottom is golden and the top is set. Flip and cook for 20 seconds. Transfer to a plate.
3. Repeat the steps with the remaining batter. Loosely cover the cooked crêpes with plastic wrap.
4. For the filling. Put all together the ingredients for filling in a saucepan on medium heat – flour, almond milk, cayenne, nutmeg, and pepper. Constantly whisk until thick or around 7 minutes. Remove from the stove. Stir in a tablespoon of parsley and cheese. Loosely cover to keep warm.
5. Spray a skillet using non-stick cooking spray and put over medium heat. Cook the garlic and mushrooms. Season with salt. Cook for 6 minutes or until the mushrooms are soft. Add 2 tablespoons of sherry. Cook for a couple of minutes. Remove from the stove. Add the remaining parsley and stir.
6. Put the crêpes side by side on a flat surface. Spread a tablespoon of the sauce and 2 tablespoons of the cooked mushrooms. Roll up the crêpes and transfer them to a greased baking dish. Put all the sauce on top. Bake in the oven at 450°F for 15 minutes.

Nutrition: Calories: 232 kcal Protein: 16.51 g Fat: 10.8 g Carbohydrates: 16.25 g

Oat Porridge with Cherry & Coconut

Preparation Time: 10 minutes

Cooking Time: 0 minutes

Servings: 3

Ingredients:

- 1 ½ cups regular oats
- 3 cups coconut almond milk
- 4 tbsp. chia seed
- 3 tbsp. raw cacao
- Coconut shavings
- Dark chocolate shavings
- Fresh or frozen tart cherries
- A pinch of stevia, optional
- Maple syrup, to taste (optional)

Directions:

1. Combine the oats, almond milk, stevia, and cacao in a medium saucepan over medium heat and bring to a boil. Lower the heat, then simmer until the oats are cooked to desired doneness.
2. Divide the porridge among 3 serving bowls and top with dark chocolate and coconut shavings, cherries, and a little drizzle of maple syrup.

Nutrition: Calories: 343 kcal Protein: 15.64 g Fat: 12.78 g Carbohydrates: 41.63 g

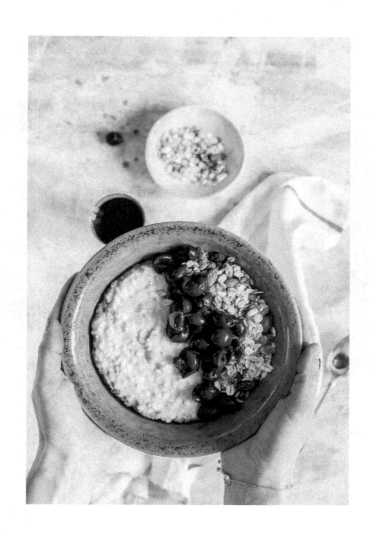

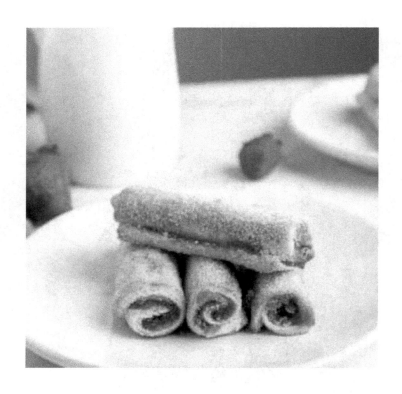

Preparation Time: 10 minutes

Cooking Time: 0 minutes

Servings: 4

Ingredients:

- 1 cup steel-cut oats
- 4 cups drinking water
- Organic Maple syrup, to taste
- 1 tsp ground cloves
- 1 ½ tbsp. ground cinnamon
- 1/8 tsp nutmeg
- ¼ tsp ground ginger
- ¼ tsp ground coriander
- ¼ tsp ground allspice
- ¼ tsp ground cardamom
- Fresh mixed berries

Directions:

1. Cook the oats based on the package instructions. When it comes to a boil, reduce heat and simmer.
2. Stir in all the spices and continue cooking until cooked to desired doneness.
3. Serve in four serving bowls and drizzle with maple syrup and top with fresh berries.
4. Enjoy!

Nutrition: Calories: 87 kcal Protein: 5.82 g Fat: 3.26 g Carbohydrates: 18.22 g

SNACKS

Rosemary and White Bean Dip

Preparation time: 10 minutes

Cooking time: 10 minutes

Servings: 10 (¼ cup per serving)

Ingredients:

- 1 (15-ounce) can cannellini beans, rinsed and drained

- 2 tablespoons extra-virgin olive oil

- 1 garlic clove, peeled

- 1 teaspoon finely chopped fresh rosemary

- Pinch cayenne pepper

- Freshly ground black pepper

- 1 (7.5-ounce) jar marinated artichoke hearts, drained

1. Blend the beans, oil, garlic, rosemary, cayenne pepper, and black pepper in a food processor until smooth.

2. Add the artichoke hearts, and pulse until roughly chopped but not puréed.

Nutrition: Calories: 75; Total Fat: 5g; Saturated Fat: 1g; Cholesterol: 0mg; Sodium: 139mg; Carbohydrates: 6g; Fiber: 3g; Added Sugars: 0g; Protein: 2g; Potassium: 75mg; Vitamin K: 1mcg

Garlicky Cale Chips

Preparation time: 5 minutes

Cooking time: 25 minutes

Servings: 4

Ingredients:

- 1 bunch curly kale

- 2 teaspoons extra-virgin olive oil

- ¼ teaspoon kosher salt

- ¼ teaspoon garlic powder (optional)

1. Preheat the oven to 325°F. Line a rimmed baking sheet with parchment paper.

2. Remove the tough stems from the kale, and tear the leaves into squares about big potato chips (they'll shrink when cooked).

3. Transfer the kale to a large bowl, and drizzle with the oil. Massage with your fingers for 1 to 2 minutes to coat well. Spread out on the baking sheet.

4. Cook for 8 minutes, then toss and cook for another 7 minutes and check them. Take them out as soon as they feel crispy, likely within the next 5 minutes.

5. Sprinkle with salt and garlic powder (if using). Enjoy immediately.

Nutrition: Calories: 28; Total Fat: 2g; Saturated Fat: 0g; Cholesterol: 0mg; Sodium: 126mg; Carbohydrates: 2g; Fiber: 1g; Added Sugars: 0g; Protein: 1g; Potassium: 81mg; Vitamin K: 114mcg

Baked Tortilla Chips

Preparation time: 5 minutes

Cooking time: 20 minutes

Servings: 4

Ingredients:

- 1 tablespoon canola or sunflower oil

- 4 medium whole-wheat tortillas

- 1/8 teaspoon coarse salt

1. Preheat the oven to 350°F.

2. Brush the oil onto both sides of each tortilla. Stack them on a large cutting board, and cut the entire stack at once, cutting the stack into 8 wedges of each tortilla. Transfer the tortilla pieces to a rimmed baking sheet. Sprinkle a little salt over each chip.

3. Bake for 10 minutes, and then flip the chips. Bake for another 3 to 5 minutes, until they're just starting to brown.

Nutrition: Calories: 194; Total Fat: 11g; Saturated Fat: 2g; Cholesterol: 0mg; Sodium: 347mg; Carbohydrates: 20g; Fiber: 4g; Added Sugars: 0g; Protein: 4g; Potassium: 111mg; Vitamin K: 7mcg

Spicy Guacamole

Preparation time: 15 minutes

Cooking time: 15 minutes

Servings: 4 (about 3 tablespoons per serving)

Ingredients:

- 1½ tablespoons freshly squeezed lime juice

- 1 tablespoon minced jalapeño pepper, or to taste

- 1 tablespoon minced red onion

- 1 tablespoon chopped fresh cilantro

- 1 garlic clove, minced

- 1/8 to ¼ teaspoon kosher salt

- Freshly ground black pepper

1. Combine the lime juice, jalapeño, onion, cilantro, garlic, salt, and pepper in a large bowl, and mix well.

Nutrition: Calories: 61; Total Fat: 5g; Saturated Fat: 1g; Cholesterol: 0mg; Sodium: 123mg; Carbohydrates: 4g; Fiber: 2g; Added Sugars: 0g; Protein: 1g; Potassium: 195mg; Vitamin K: 8mcg

Chickpea Fatteh

Preparation time: 25 minutes

Cooking time: 25 minutes

Servings: 8

Ingredients:

- 2 (4-inch) whole-wheat pitas

- 4 tablespoons extra-virgin olive oil, divided

- 1 (15-ounce) can no-salt-added chickpeas, rinsed and drained

- 1/3 cup pine nuts

- 1 cup plain 1% yogurt

- 2 garlic cloves, minced

- ¼ teaspoon salt

- ½ cup pomegranate seeds (optional)

Directions:

1. Preheat the oven to 375°F.

2. Cut the pitas into 1-inch squares (no need to separate the two halves), and toss with 2 tablespoons of oil in a large bowl. Spread onto a rimmed baking sheet and bake, occasionally shaking the sheet until golden brown, about 10 minutes.

3. Meanwhile, gently warm the chickpeas and 1 tablespoon of oil in a small saucepan over medium-low heat, 4 to 5 minutes.

4. Toast the pine nuts in a skillet with the remaining 1 tablespoon of oil over medium heat until golden brown, 4 to 5 minutes.

5. Mix the yogurt with the garlic and salt in a small bowl.

6. Transfer the toasted pitas to a wide serving bowl. Top with the chickpeas. Drizzle with the yogurt mixture, then top with the pine nuts and pomegranate seeds (if using).

Nutrition: Calories: 198; Total Fat: 12g; Saturated Fat: 2g; Cholesterol: 2mg; Sodium: 144mg; Carbohydrates: 18g; Fiber: 3g; Added Sugars: 0g; Protein: 6g; Potassium: 236mg; Vitamin K: 9mcg

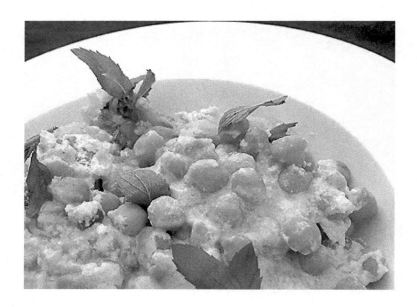

SOUP AND STEW

Amazing Zucchini Soup

Preparation Time: 10 minutes

Cooking Time: 20 minutes

Servings: 4

Ingredients:

- 1 onion, chopped

- 3 zucchinis, cut into medium chunks

- 2 tablespoons coconut almond milk

- 2 garlic cloves, minced

- 4 cups chicken stock

- 2 tablespoons coconut oil

- Pinch of salt

- Black pepper to taste

Directions:

1. Take a pot and place over medium heat.

2. Add oil and let it heat up.

3. Add zucchini, garlic, onion and stir.

4. Cook for 5 minutes.

5. Add stock, salt, pepper and stir.

6. Bring to a boil and reduce the heat.

7. Simmer for 20 minutes.

8. Remove from heat and add coconut almond milk.

9. Use an immersion blender until smooth.

10. Ladle into soup bowls and serve.

11. Enjoy!

Nutrition: Calories: 160 Fat: 2g Carbohydrates: 4g Protein: 7g Phosphorus: 110mg Potassium: 117mg Sodium: 75mg

Creamy Broccoli Cheese Salad

Preparation Time: 10 minutes

Cooking Time: 5 minutes

Servings: 8

Ingredients:

- 6 cups broccoli florets, chopped
- 1/2 cup cheddar cheese, shredded
- 3 bacon, cooked and chopped
- 1/2 tsp parsley
- 1 tsp garlic powder
- 1 tsp onion powder
- 1 1/2 tsp dill
- 1/2 cup sour cream
- 3/4 cup mayonnaise
- Pepper
- Salt

Directions:

1. Add all ingredients into the large mixing bowl and mix everything well.
2. Season salad with pepper and salt.
3. Serve and enjoy.

Nutrition: Calories 210 Fat 15.9 g Carbohydrates 11.2 g Sugar 2.8 g Protein 7.1 g Cholesterol 27 mg Phosphorus: 210mg Potassium: 217mg Sodium: 75mg

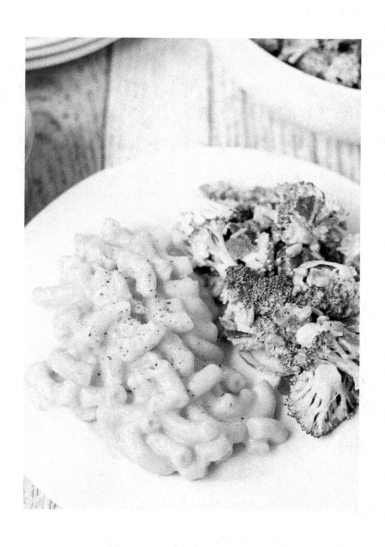

Healthy Green lettuce Salad

Preparation Time: 10 minutes

Cooking Time: 5 minutes

Servings: 4

Ingredients:

- 5 oz. fresh green lettuce
- 3 tbsp. almonds, toasted and sliced
- 1 small onion, sliced
- 1/3 cup feta cheese, crumbled
- 1 apple, sliced
- For dressing:
- 2 tsp Dijon mustard
- 1/2 tsp garlic, minced
- 3 tbsp. vinegar
- 1/3 cup olive oil
- Pepper
- Salt

Directions:

1. In a small bowl, whisk together all dressing ingredients and set aside.
2. Add green lettuce, almonds, onion, feta cheese, and apple into the large bowl and mix well.

3. Pour dressing over salad and toss well.

4. Serve and enjoy.

Nutrition: Calories 252 Fat 22.1 g Carbohydrates 12.5 g Sugar 7.5 g Protein 4.2 g Cholesterol 11 mg Phosphorus: 110mg Potassium: 117mg Sodium: 75mg

Green lettuce Strawberry Salad

Preparation Time: 10 minutes

Cooking Time: 5 minutes

Servings: 4

Ingredients:

- **For salad:**
- 6 cups baby green lettuce
- 1/4 cup walnuts, toasted and chopped
- 2.5 oz. feta cheese, crumbled
- 1 apple, cored and chopped
- 1/2 cup strawberries, sliced
- 1 1/2 cup cucumbers, sliced
- **For dressing:**
- 1 tbsp. Dijon mustard
- 1 tbsp. apple cider vinegar
- 1/4 cup olive oil
- Pepper
- Salt

Directions:

1. Add all salad ingredients into the large bowl and mix well.

2. In a small bowl, whisk together all dressing ingredients and pour over salad.

3. Toss well and serve.

Nutrition: Calories 258 Fat 21.5 g Carbohydrates 13.9 g Sugar 8.4 g Protein 6.4 g Cholesterol 16 mg Phosphorus: 120mg Potassium: 137mg Sodium: 45mg

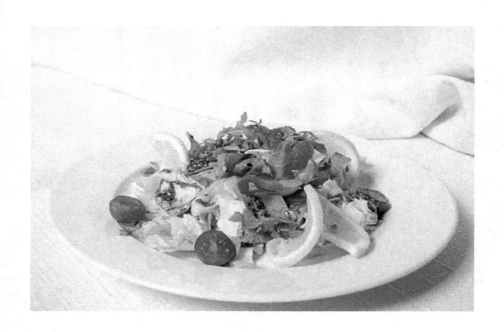

VEGETABLE

Pasta Fagioli

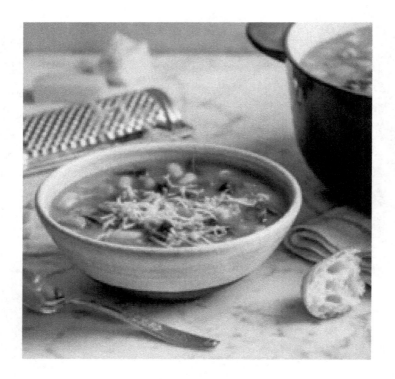

Preparation Time: 25 minutes

Cooking Time: 25 minutes

Servings: 6

Ingredients:

- 1 (15-ounce) can low-sodium great northern beans, drained and rinsed, divided

- 2 cups frozen peppers and onions, thawed, divided

- 5 cups low-sodium vegetable broth

- 1/8 teaspoon salt

- 1/8 teaspoon freshly ground black pepper

- 1 cup whole-grain orecchiette pasta

- 2 tablespoons extra-virgin olive oil

- 1/3 cup grated Parmesan cheese

Directions:

1. In a large saucepan, place the beans and cover with water. Bring to a boil over high heat and boil for 10 minutes. Drain the beans.

2. In a food processor or blender, combine 1/3 cup of beans and 1/3 cup of thawed peppers and onions. Process until smooth.

3. In the same saucepan, combine the pureed mixture, the remaining 12/3 cups of peppers and onions, the remaining beans, the broth, and the salt and pepper and bring to a simmer.

4. Add the pasta to the saucepan. Make sure to stir it and bring it to boil, reduce the heat to low, and simmer for 8 to 10 minutes, or until the pasta is tender.

5. Serve drizzled with olive oil and topped with Parmesan cheese.

Nutrition: Calories: 245 Total fat: 7g Saturated fat: 2g Sodium: 269mg Phosphorus: 188mg Potassium: 592mg Carbohydrates: 36g Fiber: 7g Protein: 12g Sugar: 4g

Roasted Peach Open-Face Sandwich

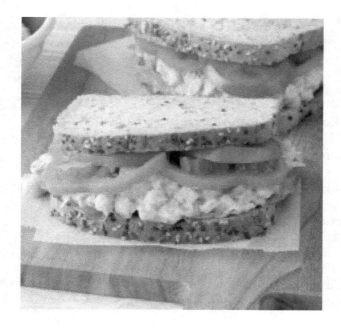

Preparation Time: 5 minutes

Cooking Time: 15 minutes

Servings: 4

Ingredients:

- 2 fresh peaches, peeled and sliced
- 1 tablespoon of extra-virgin olive oil
- 1 tablespoon of freshly squeezed lemon juice
- 1/8 teaspoon of salt
- 1/8 teaspoon of freshly ground black pepper
- 4 ounces of cream cheese, at room temperature
- 2 teaspoons of fresh thyme leaves
- 4 bread slices

Directions:

1. Preheat the oven to 400°F.

2. Arrange the peaches on a rimmed baking sheet. Brush them with olive oil on both sides.

3. Roast the peaches for 10 to 15 minutes, until they are lightly golden brown around the edges. Sprinkle with lemon juice, salt, and pepper.

4. In a small bowl, combine the cream cheese and thyme and mix well.

5. Toast the bread. Get the toasted bread and spread it with the cream cheese mixture. Top with the peaches and serve.

Nutrition: Calories: 250 Total fat: 13g Saturated fat: 6g Sodium: 376mg Phosphorus: 163mg Potassium: 260mg Carbohydrates: 28g Fiber: 3g Protein: 6g Sugar: 8g

Spicy Corn and Rice Burritos

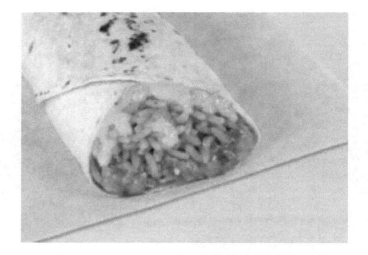

Preparation Time: 10 minutes

Cooking Time: 20 minutes

Servings: 4

Ingredients:

- 3 tablespoons of extra-virgin olive oil, divided

- 1 (10-ounce) package of frozen cooked rice

- 1½ cups of frozen yellow corn

- 1 tablespoon of chili powder

- 1 cup of shredded pepper jack cheese

- 4 large or 6 small corn tortillas

Directions:

1. Put the skillet in over medium heat and put 2 tablespoons of olive oil. Add the rice, corn, and chili powder and cook for 4 to 6 minutes, or until the ingredients are hot.

2. Transfer the ingredients from the pan into a medium bowl. Let cool for 15 minutes.

3. Stir the cheese into the rice mixture.

4. Heat the tortillas using the directions from the package to make them pliable. Fill the corn tortillas with the rice mixture, then roll them up.

5. At this point, you can serve them as is, or you can fry them first. Heat the remaining tablespoon of olive oil in a large skillet. Fry the burritos, seam-side down at first, turning once, until they are brown and crisp, about 4 to 6 minutes per side, then serve.

Nutrition: Calories: 386 Total fat: 21g Saturated fat: 7g Sodium: 510mg Phosphorus: 304mg Potassium: 282mg Carbohydrates: 41g Fiber: 4g Protein: 11g Sugar: 2g

SIDE DISHES

Garlic Cauliflower Rice

Preparation Time: 10 minutes

Cooking Time: 5 minutes

Servings: 8

Ingredients:

- 1 medium head cauliflower
- 1 tablespoon extra-virgin olive oil
- 4 garlic cloves, minced
- Freshly ground black pepper

Directions:

1. Using a sharp knife, remove the core of the cauliflower, and separate the cauliflower into florets.
2. In a food processor, pulse the florets until they are the size of rice, being careful not to over process them to the point of becoming mushy.
3. In a large skillet over medium heat, heat the olive oil. Add the garlic, and stir until just fragrant.
4. Add the cauliflower, stirring to coat. Add 1 tablespoon of water to the pan, cover, and reduce the heat to low. Steam for 7 to 10 minutes, until the cauliflower is tender. Season with pepper and serve.

Nutrition: Calories: 37; Total Fat: 2g; Saturated Fat: 0g; Cholesterol: 0mg; Carbohydrates: 4g; Fiber: 2g; Protein: 2g; Phosphorus: 35mg; Potassium: 226mg; Sodium: 22mg

Ginger Cauliflower Rice

Preparation Time: 10 minutes

Cooking Time: 10 minutes

Servings: 4

Ingredients:

- 5 cups cauliflower florets
- 3 tablespoons coconut oil
- 4 ginger slices, grated
- 1 tablespoon coconut vinegar
- 3 garlic cloves, minced
- 1 tablespoon chives, minced
- A pinch of sea salt
- Black pepper to taste

Directions:

1. Put cauliflower florets in a food processor and pulse well.
2. Heat up a pan with the oil over medium-high heat, add ginger, stir and cook for 3 minutes.
3. Add cauliflower rice and garlic, stir and cook for 7 minutes.
4. Add salt, black pepper, vinegar, and chives, stir, cook for a few seconds more, divide between plates and serve.
5. Enjoy!

Nutrition: Calories 125, fat 10,4, fiber 3,2, carbs 7,9, protein 2,7
Phosphorus: 110mg Potassium: 117mg Sodium: 75mg

SALAD

Fruity zucchini salad

Preparation time: 5 minutes

Cooking time: 5 minutes

Servings: 4 servings

Ingredients:

- 400g zucchini
- 1 small onion
- 4 tbsp. olive oil
- 100g pineapple preserve, drained
- Salt, paprika
- thyme

Directions:

1. Dice the onions and sauté in the oil until translucent.
2. Cut the zucchini into slices and add. Season with salt, paprika, and thyme.
3. Let cool and mix with the cut pineapple.

Nutrition: Energy: 150kcal, Protein: 2g, Fat: 10g, Carbohydrates: 10g, Dietary fibbers: 2g, Potassium: 220mg, Calcium: 38mg, Phosphate: 24mg

FISH & SEAFOOD

Easy Salmon and Brussels sprouts

Preparation Time: 10 minutes

Cooking Time: 10 minutes

Servings: 6

Ingredients:

- 6 deboned medium salmon fillets

- 1 tsp. onion powder

- 1 ¼ lbs. halved Brussels sprouts

- 3 tbsps. Extra virgin extra virgin olive oil

- 2 tbsps. Brown sugar

- 1 tsp. garlic powder

- 1 tsp. smoked paprika

Directions:

1. In a bowl, mix sugar with onion powder, garlic powder, smoked paprika as well as a number of tablespoon olive oil and whisk well.

2. Spread Brussels sprouts about the lined baking sheet, drizzle the rest in the essential extra virgin olive oil, toss to coat, introduce in the oven at 450 0F and bake for 5 minutes.

3. Add salmon fillets brush with sugar mix you've prepared, introduce inside the oven and bake for 15 minutes more.

4. Divide everything between plates and serve.

5. Enjoy!

Nutrition: Calories: 212, Fat: 5 g, Carbs: 12 g, Protein: 8 g, Sugars: 3.7 g, Sodium: 299.1 mg

Salmon in Dill Sauce

Preparation Time: 10 minutes

Cooking Time: 10 minutes

Servings: 6

Ingredients:

- 6 salmon fillets
- 1 c. low-fat, low-sodium chicken broth
- 1 tsp. cayenne pepper
- 2 tbsps. Fresh lemon juice
- 2 c. water
- ¼ c. chopped fresh dill

Directions:

1. In a slow cooker, mix together water, broth, lemon juice, lemon juice and dill.
2. Arrange salmon fillets on top, skin side down.
3. Sprinkle with cayenne pepper.
4. Set the slow cooker on low.
5. Cover and cook for about 1-2 hours.

Nutrition: Calories: 360, Fat: 8 g, Carbs: 44 g, Protein: 28 g, Sugars: 0.5 g, Sodium: 8 mg

Shrimp Lo Mein

Preparation Time: 10 minutes

Cooking Time: 10 minutes

Servings: 6

Ingredients:

- 1 tbsp. cornstarch

- 1 lb. medium-size frozen raw shrimp

- 1 c. frozen shelled edamame

- 3 tbsps. Light teriyaki sauce

- 16 0z. Drained and rinsed tofu spaghetti noodles

- 18 oz. frozen Szechuan vegetable blend with sesame sauce

Directions:

1. Microwave noodles for 1 minute; set aside. Place shrimp in a small bowl and toss with 2 tablespoons teriyaki sauce; set aside.

2. Place mixed vegetables and edamame in a large nonstick skillet with 1/4 cup water. Cover and cook, stirring occasionally, over medium-high heat for 7 minutes or until cooked through.

3. Stir shrimp into vegetable mixture; cover and cook 4 to 5 minutes or until shrimp is pink and cooked through.

4. Stir together remaining 1 tablespoon teriyaki sauce and the cornstarch, then stir into the mixture in the skillet until thickened. Gently stir noodles into skillet and cook until warmed through.

Nutrition: Calories: 252, Fat: 7.1 g, Carbs: 35.2 g, Protein: 12.1 g, Sugars: 2.2 g, Sodium: 180 mg

Salmon and Carrots Mix

Preparation Time: 10 minutes

Cooking Time: 10 minutes

Servings: 4

Ingredients:

- 4 oz. chopped smoked salmon

- 1 tbsp. essential olive oil

- Black pepper

- 1 tbsp. chopped chives

- ¼ c. coconut cream

- 1 ½ lbs. chopped carrots

- 2 tsps. Prepared horseradish

Directions:

1. Heat up a pan using the oil over medium heat, add carrots and cook for 10 minutes.

2. Add salmon, chives, horseradish, cream and black pepper, toss, cook for 1 minute more, divide between plates and serve.

3. Enjoy!

Nutrition: Calories: 233, Fat: 6 g, Carbs: 9 g, Protein: 11 g, Sugars: 3.3 g, Sodium: 97 mg

Smoked Salmon and Radishes

Preparation Time: 10 minutes

Cooking Time: 10 minutes

Servings: 8

Ingredients:

- ½ c. drained and chopped capers
- 1 lb. skinless, de-boned and flaked smoked salmon
- 4 chopped radishes
- 3 tbsps. Chopped chives
- 3 tbsps. Prepared beet horseradish
- 2 tsps. Grated lemon zest
- 1/3 c. roughly chopped red onion

Directions:

1. In a bowl, combine the salmon while using the beet horseradish, lemon zest, radish, capers, onions and chives, toss and serve cold.

2. Enjoy!

Nutrition: Calories: 254, Fat: 2 g, Carbs: 7 g, Protein: 7 g, Sugars: 1.4 g, Sodium: 660 mg

POULTRY RECIPES

Cilantro Drumsticks

Preparation Time: 12 minutes

Cooking Time: 18 minutes

Servings: 4

Ingredients:

- 8 chicken drumsticks
- ½ cup chimichurri sauce
- ¼ cup lemon juice

Directions:

1. Coat the chicken drumsticks with chimichurri sauce and refrigerate in an airtight container for no less than an hour, ideally overnight.
2. When it's time to cook, pre-heat your fryer to 400°F.
3. Remove the chicken from refrigerator and allow return to room temperature for roughly twenty minutes.
4. Cook for eighteen minutes in the fryer. Drizzle with lemon juice to taste and enjoy.

Nutrition: Calories: 483 Fat: 29 g Carbs: 16 g Protein: 36 g Calcium 38mg, Phosphorous 146mg, Potassium 227mg Sodium: 121 mg

Basil Chicken over Macaroni

Preparation Time: 10 minutes

Cooking Time: 30 minutes

Servings: 4

Ingredients:

- 1 (8 ounces) package macaroni
- 2 teaspoons olive oil
- 1/2 cup finely chopped onion
- 1 clove garlic, chopped
- 2 cups boneless chicken breast halves, cooked and cubed
- 1/4 cup chopped fresh basil
- 1/4 cup Parmesan cheese
- 1/2 teaspoon black pepper

Directions:

1. In a large pot of boiling water, cook macaroni until it is al dente, about 8 to 10 minutes. Drain, and set aside.

2. In a large skillet, heat oil over medium-high heat. Sauté the onions and garlic. Stir in the chicken, basil, and pepper.

3. Reduce heat to medium, and cover skillet. Simmer for about 5 minutes, stirring frequently,

4. Toss sauce with hot cooked macaroni to coat. Serve with Parmesan cheese.

Nutrition: Calories 349, Sodium 65mg, Dietary Fiber 2.2g, Total Sugars 2.1g, Protein 28.5g, Calcium 44mg, Potassium 286mg, Phosphorus 280 mg

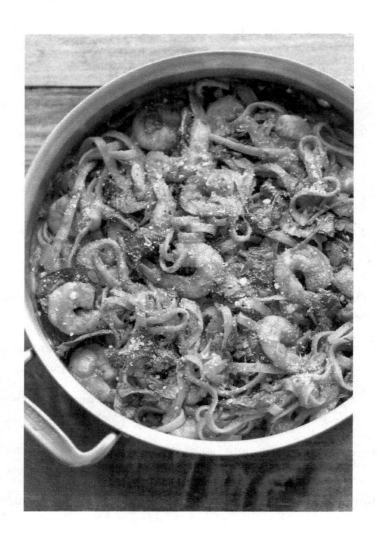

Chicken Saute

Preparation Time: 10 minutes

Cooking Time: 25 minutes

Servings: 2

Ingredients:

- 4 oz. chicken fillet
- 4 Red bell peppers, peeled
- 1 bell pepper, chopped
- 1 teaspoon olive oil
- 1 cup of water
- 1 teaspoon salt
- 1 chili pepper, chopped
- ½ teaspoon saffron

Directions:

1. Pour water in the pan and bring it to boil.
2. Meanwhile, chop the chicken fillet.
3. Add the chicken fillet in the boiling water and cook it for 10 minutes or until the chicken is tender.
4. After this, put the chopped bell pepper and chili pepper in the skillet.
5. Add olive oil and roast the vegetables for 3 minutes.
6. Add chopped Red bell peppers and mix up well.
7. Cook the vegetables for 2 minutes more.
8. Then add salt and a ¾ cup of water from chicken.
9. Add chopped chicken fillet and mix up.
10. Cook the saute for 10 minutes over the medium heat.

Nutrition: Calories 192, Fat 7.2 g, Fiber 3.8 g, Carbs 14.4 g, Protein 19.2 g Calcium 79mg, Phosphorous 216mg, Potassium 227mg Sodium: 101 mg

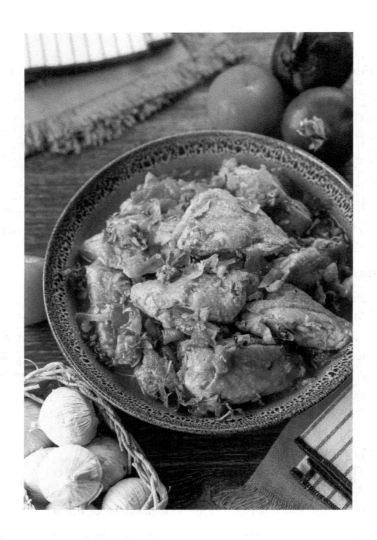

MEAT RECIPES

Grilled Lamb Chops with Fresh Mint

Preparation time: 15 min

Cooking Time: 10 minutes

Servings: 4

Ingredients:

- 8 (5 ounces) lamb loin chops, about 1 1/4-inches thick

- 1/8 teaspoon seasoning salt

- 1/2 tablespoon dried parsley

- 1/2 tablespoon minced fresh mint

- 1/2 tablespoon dried rosemary

Directions:

1. Trim any excess fat down to 1/8-inch around each lamb chop and sprinkle both sides with seasoning salt.

2. Let sit for about 30 minutes to come to room temperature.

3. Preheat an outdoor grill to 400 degrees F. Lightly oil the grate once the grill is hot.

4. Place lamb chops on the hot grate and grill for 2 to 3 minutes.

5. Rotate chops, to achieve crisscross grill marks, and continue grilling, 2 to 3 more minutes.

6. Flip the chops and grill for 2 to 3 minutes.

7. Rotate chops and continue grilling an additional 2 minutes, or until they have reached the desired doneness.

8. An instant-read thermometer inserted into the center should read at least 130 degrees F.

9. Remove chops from grill and sprinkle with dried herbs and fresh mint.

10. Allow to rest under the foil, about 10 minutes

Nutrition: Calories 160, Total Fat 6.3g, Saturated Fat 2.3g, Cholesterol 77mg, Sodium 139mg, Total Carbohydrate 0.4g, Dietary Fiber 0.2g, Total Sugars 0g, Protein 23.9g, Calcium 18mg, Iron 2mg, Potassium 295mg, Phosphorus 140mg

Lamb Keema

Preparation time: 5 min

Cooking Time: 20 minutes

Servings: 4

Ingredients:

- 1 1/2 pounds ground lamb
- 1 onion, finely chopped
- 2 teaspoons garlic powder
- 2 tablespoons garam masala
- 1/8 teaspoon salt
- 3/4 cup chicken broth

Directions:

1. In a large, heavy skillet over medium heat, cook ground lamb until evenly brown.

2. While cooking, break apart with a wooden spoon until crumbled.

3. Transfer cooked lamb to a bowl and drain off all but 1 tablespoon fat. Saute onion until soft and translucent, about 5 minutes.

4. Stir in garlic powder, and sauté 1 minute.

5. Stir in garam masala and cook 1 minute.

6. Return the browned lamb to the pan, and stir in chicken beef broth.

7. Reduce heat, and simmer for 10 to 15 minutes or until meat is fully cooked through, and liquid has evaporated.

Nutrition: Calories 194, Total Fat 7.3g, Saturated Fat 2.6g, Cholesterol 87mg, Sodium 160mg, Total Carbohydrate 2.2g, Dietary Fiber 0.4g, Total Sugars 0.9g, Protein 28.1g, Calcium 18mg, Iron 2mg, Potassium 379mg, Phosphorus 240mg

BROTHS, CONDIMENT AND SEASONING

Butteralmond milk Herb Dressing

Preparation Time: 15 minutes

Cooking Time: 0 minutes

Servings: 1 ½ cup

Ingredients:

- ½ cup skim almond milk
- ½ cup Low-Sodium Mayonnaise
- 2 tablespoons apple cider vinegar
- ½ scallion, green part only, chopped
- 1 tablespoon chopped fresh dill
- 1 teaspoon chopped fresh thyme
- ½ teaspoon minced garlic
- Freshly ground black pepper

Directions:

1. Mix the almond milk, mayonnaise, and vinegar until smooth in a medium bowl. Whisk in the scallion, dill, thyme, and garlic. Season with pepper. Store.

Nutrition: Calories: 31 Fat: 2g Sodium: 19mg Carbohydrates: 2g Phosphorus: 13mg Potassium: 26mg Protein: 0g

Poppy Seed Dressing

Preparation Time: 15 minutes

Cooking Time: 0 minutes

Servings: 2 cups

Ingredients:

- ½ cup apple cider or red wine vinegar
- 1/3 cup honey
- ¼ cup freshly squeezed lemon juice
- 1 tablespoon Dijon mustard
- 1 cup olive oil
- ½ small sweet onion, minced
- 2 tablespoons poppy seeds

Directions:

1. Mix the vinegar, honey, lemon juice, and mustard in a small bowl. Whisk in the oil, onion, and poppy seeds. Store the dressing in a sealed glass container in the refrigerator for up to 2 weeks.

Nutrition: Calories: 151 Fat: 14g Sodium: 12mg Carbohydrates: 7g Phosphorus: 13mg Potassium: 30mg Protein: 0g

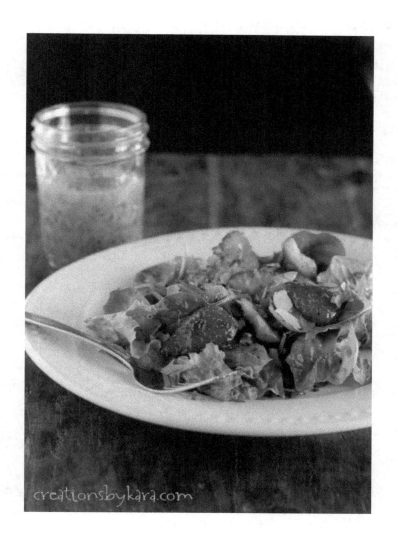

creationsbykara.com

DRINKS AND SMOOTHIES

Green Coconut Smoothie

Preparation Time: 10 minutes

Cooking Time: 3 minutes

Servings: 2

Ingredients:

- 1 1/4 cup coconut almond milk (canned)

- 2 tablespoon chia seeds

- 1 cup of fresh kale leaves

- 1 cup of green lettuce leaves

- 1 scoop vanilla protein powder

- 1 cup ice cubes

- Granulated stevia sweetener (to taste; optional)

- 1/2 cup water

Directions:

1. Rinse and clean kale and the green lettuce leaves from any dirt.

2. Add all ingredients in your blender.

3. Blend until you get a nice smoothie.

4. Serve into chilled glass.

Nutrition: Calories: 179, Carbohydrates: 5g, Proteins: 4g, Fat: 18g, Fiber: 2.5g Calcium 22mg, Phosphorous 46mg, Potassium 34mg Sodium: 131 mg

Fruity Smoothie

Preparation Time: 10minutes

Cooking Time: 0 minutes

Servings: 2

Ingredients:

- 8 oz. canned fruits, with juice
- 2 scoops vanilla-flavored whey protein powder
- 1 cup cold water
- 1 cup crushed ice

Directions:

1. First, start by putting all the ingredients in a blender jug.
2. Give it a pulse for 30 seconds until blended well.
3. Serve chilled and fresh.

Nutrition: Calories 186 Protein 23 g Fat 2g Cholesterol 41 mg Potassium 282 mg Calcium 160 mg Fiber 1.1 g

DESSERT

Blueberry espresso brownies

Preparation time: 15 minutes

Cooking time: 30 minutes

Servings: 12

Ingredients:

- 1/4 cup organic cocoa powder
- 1/4 teaspoon salt
- 1/2 cup raw honey
- 1/2 teaspoon baking soda
- 1 cup blueberries
- 1 cup coconut cream
- 1 tablespoon cinnamon
- 1 tablespoon ground coffee
- 2 teaspoon vanilla extract
- 3 eggs

Directions:

1. Preheat the oven to 3250f.
2. In a bow mix together coconut cream, honey, eggs, cinnamon, honey, vanilla, baking soda, coffee and salt.

3. Use a mixer to combine all ingredients.

4. Fold in the blueberries

5. Pour the batter in a greased baking dish and bake for 30 minutes or until a toothpick inserted in the middle comes out clean.

6. Remove from the oven and let it cool.

Nutrition: Calories: 168; carbs: 20g; protein: 4g; fats: 10g; phosphorus: 79mg; potassium: 169mg; sodium: 129mg

Spiced peaches

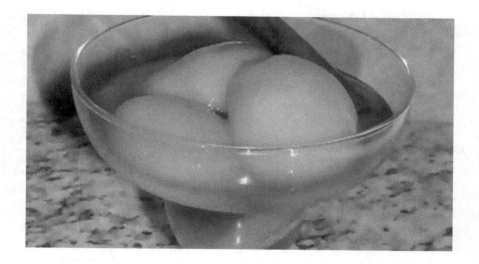

Preparation time: 5 minutes

Cooking time: 10 minutes

Servings: 2 servings

Ingredients:

- Peaches – 1 cup

- Cornstarch – ½ tsp.

- Ground cloves – 1 tsp.

- Ground cinnamon – 1 tsp.

- Ground nutmeg – 1 tsp.

- Zest of ½ lemon

- Water – ½ cup

Directions:

1. Combine cinnamon, cornstarch, nutmeg, ground cloves, and lemon zest in a pan on the stove.

2. Heat on a medium heat and add peaches.

3. Bring to a boil, reduce the heat and simmer for 10 minutes.

4. Serve.

Nutrition: calories: 70; fat: 0g; carb: 14g; phosphorus: 23mg; potassium: 176mg; sodium: 3mg; protein: 1g

Pumpkin cheesecake bar

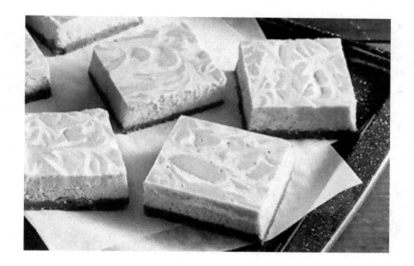

Preparation time: 10 minutes

Cooking time: 50 minutes

Servings: 4 servings

Ingredients:

- Unsalted butter – 2 ½ tbsps.

- Cream cheese – 4 oz.

- All-purpose white flour – ½ cup

- Golden brown sugar – 3 tbsps.

- Granulated sugar – ¼ cup

- Pureed pumpkin – ½ cup

- Egg whites - 2

- Ground cinnamon – 1 tsp.

- Ground nutmeg – 1 tsp.

- Vanilla extract – 1 tsp.

Directions:

1. Preheat the oven to 350f.

2. Mix flour and brown sugar in a bowl.

3. Mix in the butter to form 'breadcrumbs'.

4. Place ¾ of this mixture in a dish.

5. Bake in the oven for 15 minutes. Remove and cool.

6. Lightly whisk the egg and fold in the cream cheese, sugar, pumpkin, cinnamon, nutmeg and vanilla until smooth.

7. Pour this mixture over the oven-baked base and sprinkle with the rest of the breadcrumbs from earlier.

8. Bake in the oven for 30 to 35 minutes more.

9. Cool, slice and serve.

Nutrition: calories: 248; fat: 13g; carb: 33g; phosphorus: 67mg; potassium: 96mg; sodium: 146mg; protein: 4g

Apple crunch pie

Preparation time: 10 minutes

Cooking time: 35 minutes

Servings: 8

Ingredients

- large tart apples, peeled, seeded and sliced
- ½ cup of white all-purpose flour
- 1/3 cup margarine
- 1 cup of sugar
- ¾ cup of rolled oat flakes
- ½ teaspoon of ground nutmeg

Directions

1 Preheat the oven to 375f/180c.
2 Place the apples over a lightly greased square pan (around 7 inches).
3 Mix the rest of the ingredients in a medium bowl with and spread the batter over the apples.
4 Bake for 30-35 minutes or until the top crust has gotten golden brown.
5 Serve hot.

Nutrition: Calories: 261.9 kcal Carbohydrate: 47.2 g Protein: 1.5 g Sodium: 81 mg Potassium: 123.74 mg Phosphorus: 35.27 mg Dietary fiber: 2.81 g Fat: 7.99 g

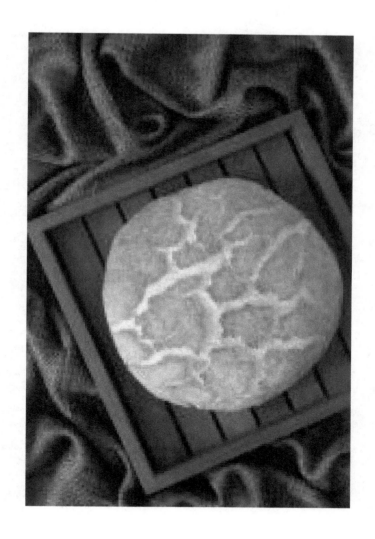

CPSIA information can be obtained
at www.ICGtesting.com
Printed in the USA
LVHW080027240321
682294LV00009B/797